CW00552552

NUTRITION

EXPLAINED

The Facts

Kathleen Gardiner

First published in the UK 2015
by Nutritional Wisdom Publishing

e-mail: info@nwpublishing.co.uk

Copyright c 2015 Kathleen Gardiner
Illustrations copyright c 2015 Kathleen Gardiner

The moral right of the author has been asserted

All rights reserved. No part of this publication may be reproduced
or transmitted in any form or by any means, electronic,
mechanical, photocopying, recording or by any information
storage or retrievable system, without the prior permission of the
publisher.

ISBN: 978-0-9557357-4-5

Printed by A1 Press, Dryson House, York Industrial Estate, York
Road, Wetherby, LS22 7SU

FOOD FOR THOUGHT

The power of food blows my mind, as does the complex infra-structure of the human body which would not exist without the lifeblood of the food system. It cannot be denied that the grand plan has been adapted to the multiplication of life on earth.

How can anyone not believe in a higher power?

Contents

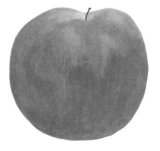

He who ignores the powers of nutrition wastes the time of the physician
(Old Chinese Proverb)

INTRODUCTION

Nutrition is a complex science. Perhaps for this reason and the fact that we are constantly bombarded with what we should and should not eat, we unfortunately turn off from the reality and the importance of healthy eating.

My theory is that key, basic messages of nutrition are unlikely to sink in unless we are informed, in an uncomplicated way, of the reasons WHY some foods are beneficial to our health and others are not. I have addressed this in a step by step approach.

Firstly, my aim is to highlight salient facts that will surprise and benefit you without the confusion of technical jargon. Secondly, to suggest ways which may help you think *differently* about food and thirdly, to provide a 'Reference Guide' and explanation of all the major vitamins and specific food groups. I do not intend to swamp your mind with scientific data, charts or figures.

You will be surprised how understanding the basics can change your life.

It is not easy to adopt a new 'Conscious Eating' lifestyle. However, once you have trained your brain to think '*differently*' about the foods you eat, you will then begin to accept, by choice, a different eating lifestyle. When you know the basics you are armed with the fundamental, nutritional knowledge that will hopefully become the cornerstone of your every day eating regime. Eating nutrient rich food is a real pleasure.

I am confident that if you are serious about making a difference to your wellbeing and lifestyle, this guide-book will have a positive impact on your choice.

-0-0-0-

The aim of this book is to provide information on diet and nutrients. The contents are not intended to offer personal medical advice. Never disregard professional medical advice or delay in seeking it because of something you have read in this book.

Good nutrition is a pathway to the prevention of illness, not a cure. If you have an existing health problem, including allergies or mal-absorption problems, you must consult your doctor. However, in times of ill health nutrition is your best friend.

-0-0-0-

A Journal has been included at the back of this guide-book. You may find it useful.

He who ignores the powers of nutrition wastes the time of the physician
(Old Chinese Proverb)

PART 1

THE GOOD GUYS

He who ignores the powers of nutrition wastes the time of the physician
(Old Chinese Proverb)

Chapter 1

MOTHER NATURE'S ARMY

Our bodies are made up of trillions of cells, often referred to as the 'Building Blocks of Life'. If we do not keep our cells healthy they will become diseased, causing us to become unwell and, at worst, may give rise to developing serious, life threatening conditions.

From the onset think of nutrients in food as 'Mother Nature's Army'. Think of your body as a fortress and the food you eat as an army, protecting the fortress.

To keep our cells healthy we need to nourish them on a daily basis with ANTIOXIDANTS. These substances are contained in the vitamins abundant in all fruits and vegetables. Antioxidants are vital in the war against FREE RADICALS (See Chapter 5). For the moment think of ANTIOXIDANTS as the good guys and FREE RADICALS as the bad guys.

ANTIOXIDANTS

MOTHER NATURE'S GENERALS

Although our bodies produce their own antioxidants, we also need to boost our defences by eating antioxidant rich fruit and vegetables, which provide beta-carotene, vitamins B, C, E & K to help maintain a healthy immune system.

Fruit and Vegetables with a deep colour, including dark green leafy vegetables, peppers, carrots and tomatoes, are particularly rich in beta-carotene which the body can convert into vitamin A. If eaten raw you can be sure to optimise on their powerful health benefits, hence the saying, 'Raw Energy'. Tomatoes, however, release more of their antioxidant, 'Lycopene', when cooked in a little olive oil. Most fruits and berries, particularly blueberries, cranberries and cherries are major sources of antioxidants.

The following chapter deals with the individual antioxidant rich vitamins, the beating heart of the healthy eating message. This is a very useful reference guide.

He who ignores the powers of nutrition wastes the time of the physician
(Old Chinese Proverb)

Chapter 2

VITAMINS – THE ARMED FORCES

Water Soluble Vitamins

I recently conducted an independent survey, which proved that a high majority of people are not aware of which vitamins are water soluble and those which are fat soluble. It also proved that few people know what free radicals and antioxidants really are. This was the tipping point which prompted me to write this guide-book and explains the importance of basic nutritional knowledge.

It is important that you are aware that vitamin 'C' and the family of eight 'B' vitamins are water soluble. This is because any excess of these vitamins leaves your body via your waterworks and sweat. Your body will not store these vitamins. Therefore, it is advisable to ingest foods containing water soluble vitamins daily to achieve optimum health. Their specific health properties are given below.

(All other vitamins are fat soluble which means that any excess is stored in your liver, sometimes for up to six months. This is why we refer to the liver as being the 'Power House of the Body'. It is also the reason why fat soluble vitamin supplements should not be necessary unless you have a vitamin absorption problem, with the exception of vitamin D).

Here are some facts about the water soluble vitamins..

VITAMIN 'C' (ascorbic acid)

Vitamin C is vital for the maintenance of healthy connective tissue which is made up of collagen and elastin. It works by uniting the muscle fibres into bundles and supports the blood vessels, like a kind of soft skeleton. We must obtain our vitamin C from food as the body is unable to form any of its own. Deficiency would soon result in bleeding, especially from small blood vessels under the skin and from the gums. Wounds would heal more slowly. Scurvey would follow and, if the deficiency is prolonged, death would result. However, excessively high intakes can lead to diarrhoea in some people.

Adequate intake of Vitamin C has been shown to be helpful in reducing the severity of conditions like osteoarthritis, rheumatoid arthritis and asthma, and for preventing conditions such as colon cancer, atherosclerosis and heart disease. It may also be useful for preventing recurrent ear infections.

Almost all our vitamin C is derived from fruit and vegetables, (small amounts are present in milk and liver). Unfortunately, this vitamin is, perhaps, the least stable of all the vitamins; it can soon be lost during storage, preparation and cooking.

The best method of cooking vegetables is to steam them, thereby less vitamin C is lost. Also the fresher your fruit and vegetables, the more vitamin C they contain. We, as a nation, must eat more fruits and vegetables to maintain daily healthy levels of water soluble vitamins.

Some more interesting facts about Vitamin C....

- Vitamin C is a 'Major Antioxidant' and 'Fat Blaster' vitamin. Most fruits contain Vitamin C but the richest source is found in citrus fruits such as oranges, tangerines, lemons, limes and grapefruits. Also kiwi fruit, blackcurrants and cherries.

- Vitamin C is essential for the production of collagen, healthy skin and healing of wounds.

- Vitamin C is not stable in heat. However, any juices from cooking, particularly steaming or microwaving, provide a flavoursome stock and can be frozen for later use in sauces, soups, gravies etc.,

- Kiwi fruit contains twice as much vitamin C as an equivalent amount of orange

- Red Bell Peppers are extremely rich in Vitamin C.

- Oranges and grapefruits have long been used in traditional Chinese medicine, particularly to stimulate the digestive system and treat constipation

- Lemon juice contains an oil which helps to expel toxins from the body. Try starting your day with a mug of warm, boiled water and the juice of half a fresh lemon. Strange as this may seem, it has an alkaline affect to your system (see P.80).

- Vitamin C is not a cure for the common cold but it is thought to reduce the symptoms and longevity of the cold

- IF YOU ARE A SMOKER, BEWARE!!! − Smoking inhibits the absorption of vitamin C

- Vitamin C helps the absorption of other vitamins, particularly the family of B vitamins, also the minerals zinc and iron

- Vitamin B2 and B6 are more active in the presence of vitamin C

- Vitamin C aids calcium absorption.

- Always buy firm fruits, slightly soft to the touch. These are fresher and have a denser nutrient content.

- Vitamin C may also protect the skin against free radical damage after exposure to ultraviolet rays. However, it is essential to protect your skin with a high UV factor if exposed to strong sunlight. It is particularly vital for those with pale skin, freckles and moles

- Aim to have two pieces of fruit with your breakfast e.g. A few berries, an apricot or a kiwi. Fruit is delicious with porridge and it provides a quick, healthy punch packed start to the day.

Tick any of the above tips that you think may help you, or cross-reference them in your log at the end of the book.

THE FAMILY OF EIGHT 'B' VITAMINS

THE 'BUSY BEES'

The B vitamins are also vital for our health. Sometimes referred to as 'B Complex'. Like vitamin C, this family of eight vitamins is water soluble and most are also sensitive to heat. Remember, your bodies are unable to store water soluble vitamins, therefore, a regular, daily intake is necessary. A lack of these vitamins can result in multiple deficiency diseases within a few months.

Think of the B family of vitamins as the 'Busy Bees'. The honeycomb representing the trillions of cells in your body and, like the bees, the B complex nutrients are a powerful workforce producing an energy promoting product.

Most of the B vitamins are responsible for the production of energy, helping to combat fatigue, but each one has a different method of achieving this. In addition some have other unique properties.

Due to the complexity of the eight B vitamins, rather than give you information overload at this stage, I have listed below the foods from which they can be drawn. For those wishing to learn about the unique properties, function and deficiency consequences of the individual B vitamins, these are listed in detail on page 20.

Food sources containing B vitamins: Specific B vitamins are found in one or more of these foods: milk, eggs, offal, pork, whole grains, lentils, fruits, vegetables, fortified breakfast cereals, fish including salmon, spinach, broccoli, roast chicken, whole wheat bread and peanuts. Remember, not all of the eight vitamins are contained in all of these foods.

You will have noticed that, unlike vitamin C, B Complex is found in a wide range of foods so deficiency is less likely.

THE UNIQUE PROPERTIES
&
FUNCTION OF INDIVIDUAL
B COMPLEX VITAMINS

Vitamin B1 – THIAMIN:

Thiamin is essential for boosting our cells with the continuous release of energy from carbohydrate. It is found in a wide variety of foods, including animal and vegetable foods. The richest sources are milk, eggs, offal, pork, whole grains, wholegrain breads, lentils, fruits, vegetables and fortified breakfast cereals.

Most people should be able to get all the thiamin they need from a varied and balanced diet.

Vitamin B2 – RIBOFLAVIN:

Riboflavin is essential for the utilisation of energy from food and also supports the antioxidant activity in the body. It is found in foods of animal origin such as milk and its products including yogurt, eggs, salmon and lean meats. Other good sources are Soybeans, spinach almonds, legumes and fortified breakfast cereals.

As riboflavin is destroyed by sunlight, bottled milk should not be allowed to stay too long on the doorstep. It is also worth noting that vegans have low intakes of this vitamin. Otherwise, specific deficiency signs are rarely seen but include sores in the corners of the mouth.

Vitamin B3 – NIACIN:

This vitamin is involved in the utilisation of food energy. (It is formed by two B–vitamins, nicotinic acid and nicotinamide). Deficiency results in pellagra in which the skin becomes dark and scaly, especially when exposed to light. Good sources of niacin include beef, roast chicken, fish, whole wheat bread, peanuts and lentils.

Vitamin B5 –PANTOTHENIC ACID

Pantothenic acid is necessary for the release of energy from fat and carbohydrate. Dietary deficiencies of this vitamin are unlikely because it is so widespread in food.

Vitamin B6 – PYRIDOXINE:

Involved in over 100 cellular reactions throughout the body, B6 is instrumental in keeping various bodily functions working at their best. It is involved in the metabolism of amino acids and is necessary for the formation of haemoglobin. Deficiency is rare in humans as it occurs widely in food, especially meat, fish, eggs, whole cereals and some vegetables.

Vitamin B7– BIOTIN:

Very small amounts of Biotin are essential for the metabolism of fat (i.e.to convert into energy). Studies have shown that this vitamin may help in the health of hair, skin and nails. Rich sources include offal and egg yolk. Smaller amounts are obtained from milk and dairy products, cereals, fish, fruit and vegetables.

Vitamin B12

Vitamin B12 is a mixture of several related compounds, all of which contain the trace element cobalt. Together with folate, it is needed by rapidly dividing cells such as those in the bone marrow which form blood cells. Deficiency leads to a condition known as Pernicious Anaemia.

Because vitamin B12 does not occur in vegetable foods, deficiency may occur in vegans who do not consume meat, milk, eggs or special supplements. However the more common reason for deficiency is found in those who cannot absorb this vitamin.

Sources are found in liver (the richest source), yeast, eggs, cheese, milk, meat, fish and in fortified breakfast cereals.

FOLATE:

Folate has several functions, including its action with vitamin B12 in rapidly dividing cells. Deficiency leads to a characteristic form of anaemia, which must be distinguished from that caused by a deficiency of vitamin B12.

Folate deficiency can result not only from a poor diet, but also from a) increased needs for the synthesis of red blood cells in pregnant women, b) from increased requirements arising from certain medical conditions in the elderly and c) when there is decreased absorption of folate in gastro-intestinal disease.

Pregnant women are advised to take a daily dietary supplement of folate before pregnancy and during its early stages to help reduce their risk of having a baby with spina bifida. They are also advised to eat plenty of folate rich foods during this period.

Sources occur in small amounts in many foods. Excellent sources of folate are green leafy vegetables, spinach, bok choy, parsley and romaine lettuce. Other strong sources include asparagus, cauliflower, broccoli, beets and lentils. Some fruits are important sources of folate too, such as papayas and strawberries. To a lesser degree, oranges, pineapple, raspberries, kiwifruit, lemons and limes are all 'good' sources of this vitamin.

I hope you are convinced of the reasons WHY you need to ensure that your daily diet includes sufficient Vitamin C and Vitamin B Complex. The above detailed account of the individual B vitamins may be of particular interest for those who are showing similar deficiency symptoms.

In conclusion of the water soluble vitamins, I would recommend that you eat a piece of citrus fruit or a kiwi fruit most days, particularly during the winter months. This would give you your daily GDA (Guideline Daily Amount) of vitamin C. In addition I would recommend that you start your day with a bowl of porridge made with skimmed or semi-skimmed milk or other breakfast cereal, preferably one that has no added sugar. This and a balanced diet should ensure that you have your full GDA of water-soluble vitamins.

FAT SOLUBLE VITAMINS

As explained earlier in Chapter 2, any excess of fat soluble vitamins is stored in your liver, providing your body with a storehouse to draw from. It should not be necessary to take supplements unless subscribed by a doctor due to your body being unable to absorb this vitamin in its natural form.

These vitamins are stand alone vitamins, therefore, it would be helpful for you to be aware of their individual unique properties, as listed below.

Vitamin A – RETINOL

Vitamin A itself is found only in foods of animal origin, in particular liver. However certain foods containing beta-carotene, such as deep green, yellow, orange or red fruits and vegetables can be converted in the body to 'Retinol', thereby becoming sources of vitamin A activity.

Deficiency: Vitamin A is essential for vision in dim light. Prolonged deficiency results in night blindness. This vitamin is also necessary for the maintenance of healthy skin and surface tissue.

Excessive doses which accumulate in the liver can be poisonous. Pregnant women, as a matter of precaution, are advised not to take vitamin A supplements or to eat liver, except on the advice of their doctor due to the possibility of some birth defects.

Sources: Offal, fish liver oils, dairy produce and eggs. Variable amounts of beta-carotene are found in carrots and dark green or yellow vegetables, roughly in proportion to the depth of their colour, thus dark vegetables such as spinach contain more than cabbage. All margarine for retail sale is required by law to contain about the same amount of vitamin A as butter.

Vitamin D:

Vitamin D is vital to help maintain bone health by ensuring a plentiful supply of calcium in the blood. It achieves this primarily by enhancing the absorption of dietary calcium from the intestine. Without vitamin D, little or no calcium can be absorbed.

The vitamins A and K help the absorption of vitamin D.

Sources: Sunlight is by far the most important source for most people, who will need little or no extra from food. All natural dietary sources are from animal origin, particularly fish livers. Other sources are milk products, eggs and some fortified cereals.

Most people should be able to make enough vitamin D from regular, short, casual exposure to the sun, without adding substantially to the risk of skin cancer.

You do not have to redden or burn your skin to make enough vitamin D. If you think you may be deficient, this can be determined by a simple blood test. Your doctor would prescribe a vitamin D supplement in this instance.

Vitamin E:

The major vitamin E activity in the body is as a powerful antioxidant. This vitamin occurs widely in food. Like all other fat soluble vitamins it is stored in the body, therefore, deficiencies are rarely seen. Taking supplements is not advised unless prescribed by a doctor in the event of a mal-absorption problem.

High levels of this potent antioxidant decreases the risk of a heart attack or stroke in most people.

Sources: The richest sources are found in vegetable oils, nuts and seeds, some cereal products, egg yolk and animal fats and meat. Fruit and vegetables contain comparatively little.

Vitamin K:

Vitamin K is necessary for the normal clotting of blood. It is also well established that this vitamin has a role in bone support for post menopausal women who start to experience bone loss.

Sources: Deficiency is unlikely, partly because it is widespread in vegetables such as spinach, kale, parsley, cauliflower, broccoli, brussels sprouts, cabbage, peas and cereals and partly because our intestinal bacteria can synthesise it.

He who ignores the powers of nutrition wastes the time of the physician
(Old Chinese Proverb)

Chapter 3

FIBRE

Nature's Scavengers

In addition to antioxidant rich foods helping in the war against free radicals, in my view, not enough emphasis is made of the vital role that fibre has to play in this regard. Apart from getting rid of waste matter it expels and prevents the build up of toxins in the body, aids digestion and helps prevent disease. Without fibre, toxins can play havoc with our health.

Fibre rich foods are essential for reducing the risk of many serious health conditions such as colon cancers, high blood pressure, regulating blood sugar levels, heart disease, diabetes, obesity and supporting weight loss.

There are two types of fibre, soluble and insoluble. Soluble fibre dissolves in water and forms a gel which slows down the stomach helping to keep hunger pangs at bay. Insoluble fibre does not dissolve in water.

Soluble fibre constituents which may be absorbed into the bloodstream are found especially in fruit, vegetables, nuts, seeds, oatmeal and lentils and help to reduce the amount of cholesterol in the blood. Pectin is a rich source of soluble fibre. The skin and pulp of fresh apples and citrus fruits are rich in pectin. It is believed that soluble fibre may affect blood sugar levels and have a beneficial effect on insulin sensitivity, thus helping to control diabetes.

Insoluble fibre is not absorbed into the body, instead it adds bulk to the faeces by passing through the gastrointestinal tract relatively intact, helping to speed up the waste through your gut. Apart from gathering up toxins, an additional benefit to health is that it helps to prevent constipation. Food sources of insoluble fibre include starchy foods such as potatoes, rice, grains, bread and pasta. Wholegrain varieties of starchy foods will increase the amount of fibre you are eating and particularly foods with their skins on.

He who ignores the powers of nutrition wastes the time of the physician
(Old Chinese Proverb)

Chapter 4

FRUITS AND VEGETABLES

Knights of The Food Table

The American guideline for the dietary intake of fruit and vegetables is about 50%,(approximately two pieces of different fruit per day and four or more different types of vegetables). It is possible that when the UK guidelines are reviewed in the near future, this recommendation will match that of the American guideline.

As well as vitamins, fruits and vegetables contain a wide range of other compounds with varying levels of antioxidant activity. They are also a vital source of soluble and insoluble fibre. Research is continuing into the possible role of these compounds in the prevention of heart disease, and cancer.

To help you further with the intense powers of vitamin rich foods, the following pages are devoted to 10 specific fruits and vegetables and their unique antioxidant properties, revealing what diseases they offer protection for. I believe they truly have potent health benefits which cannot help but inspire you. However, I must point out that there are many more deserving fruits and vegetables which equal most of those on the 'Top Ten' list. These are listed separately.

We are all victims of our birth and so we must look to our lineage for clues as to the possible health flaws in our genetic makeup. Look out for specific properties in the following fruits and vegetables which may help boost any genetic weakness you may have inherited.

Remember, do not overcook your vegetables. Soggy vegetables result in a loss of nutrients and a loss of flavour.

Try and buy organic whenever possible, particularly in regard to root vegetables which you use regularly, such as carrots, celery and potatoes.

I would recommend that you use the section of 'Top Ten Fruits and Vegetables' as a reference guide, to help remind you of WHY these foods are so vital for your health and wellbeing. These are listed in alphabetical order.

Keep your intake of fruits and vegetables varied and interesting.

Don't forget to make notes in your journal of any specific information which may help you.

He who ignores the powers of nutrition, wastes the time of the physician
(Old Chinese Proverb)

TOP TEN FRUITS AND VEGETABLES

<u>APPLES</u>

Apples are continually being ranked in the top ten 'Healthy Foods' and are often acclaimed as a 'miracle food'. They are extremely rich in vital antioxidants – the good guys! Also they are a great source of pectin which is dietary fibre; this helps prevent the amount of bad cholesterol in your blood from rising.

This fruit is so delicious and is readily available all year round. Their antioxidant content provides particularly strong cardiovascular and specific cancer benefits. So powerful are the plant nutrients and antioxidants in this little round fruit, they may play a big hand in reducing the risk of developing hypertension and diabetes and may also help to improve regulation of our blood sugar levels (See Page 74).

You will be amazed to realise that an apple with the skin contains the following nutrients, most of which have been explained in more detail in specific parts of the guide-book:

Vitamin C, Beta-carotene, Thiamin (Vitamin B1), Riboflavin (vitamin B2), Pantotenic Acid (Vitamin B5), Folate (Vitamin B9), Vitamins E, K and Niacin (B3), Calcium, Magnesium, Phosphorus, iron, manganese and potassium.

Apples contain almost no fat, sodium, or cholesterol and are a great source of fibre.

I would recommend that you introduce apples into your regular eating regime. A small apple is fine. Aim for at least three per week. You will also find them quite filling, so eat as a mid morning or mid afternoon snack with a few nuts, such as brazils nuts and almonds. If you cannot eat nuts have a few pumpkin seeds and/or sunflower seeds. The dietary fat content in nuts and seeds will aid the absorption of fat soluble vitamins contained in fruit and help to balance blood sugar levels. Definitely one to note down in your journal and, of course, one to put high on your weekly shopping list.

Specific Health Benefits:

- <u>Cardiovascular Benefits:</u> The cardiovascular benefits of apples are well documented in research studies. They are closely associated with two aspects of apple nutrients, their content of water-soluble fibre, pectin, and their unusual mix of plant chemicals that work as antioxidants.

- Total cholesterol including the bad cholesterol (LDL), is decreased by eating one small apple every day.

- Recent researchers believe that the antioxidant, Quercetin, content of apples also provides our cardiovascular system with anti-inflammatory benefits.

- <u>Anti-Cancer Benefits:</u> The benefits from apples, as far as lung cancer is concerned, is what excites researchers, although some preliminary results show that apples may benefit several different cancer types, especially colon cancer and breast cancer.

- <u>Anti-Asthma Benefits</u>: Multiple studies have shown apple intake to be associated with decreased risk of asthma. This benefit is definitely associated with the antioxidant and anti-inflammatory nutrients found in this fruit. However, scientists believe there is very likely to be something else going on as well, since apples appear to be a remarkable, standout fruit in regard to asthma benefits.

- <u>Other Health Benefits</u>: Preliminary health benefits of apples have also been established for several age-related health problems, including degeneration of the eyes and neurodegenerative problems, including Alzheimer's disease.

APPLE JUICE: A glass of this juice contains as much sugar as an equivalent glass of some fizzy drinks!!!
Apple juice should be diluted with approximately two thirds of water due to its high sugar content. Whole apples are a much better nutritional choice. The juice of apples does not contain any soluble fibre.

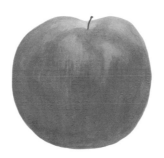

AVOCADOS

Avocados are a fruit, sometimes referred to as Alligator Pears because of their shape.

Impressive Anti-Inflammatory Benefits: According to the George Mateljan Foundation, this fruit has, unquestionably in the world of health research, the ability to help prevent inflammation. Arthritis, including osteoarthritis and rheumatoid arthritis, have received special research attention with respect to dietary intake of avocados. No single category of nutrients in avocado is more impressive than carotenoids. This fruit contains eight key carotenoid antioxidants, all providing anti-inflammatory benefits.

Cardiovascular Health: The aforesaid Foundation also report, that avocado support for heart and blood vessels might be surprising to those who think of avocado as being too high in fat for heart health. However, from a research standpoint, many metabolic aspects of heart health, including levels of inflammatory risk factors and blood fat levels (including level of total cholesterol), are improved by avocado. Moreover, it is known that heart health is improved by the intake of oleic acid, the primary fatty acid in avocado, together with the intake of omega-3 fatty acids, also contained in this amazing fruit.

Avocados are brimming with other heart-healthy nutrients, such as vitamin E, folate, potassium and monounsaturated fats.

Anti-Cancer Benefits: Research into anti-cancer benefits are showing impressive, preliminary results, particularly in the ability of avocado to help prevent the occurrence of cancers in the mouth, skin and prostate gland.

Avocados contain more potassium than bananas and are rich in folic acid, vitamin B6 and vitamin K. Other good dietary sources include complex B vitamins, vitamin C and E. Avocados are also believed to aid digestion.

Surprisingly, these potent pearls are a good source of dietary fibre.

Avocados are excellent for healthy, youthful looking skin. They maintain good levels of moisture in the epidermal layer of the skin and improve skin tone largely due to the high level of monounsaturated fat content. Other healthy skin promoting properties in avocados come from vitamin E and Vitamin C.

BEETROOT

Wow! This blockbuster vegetable and potent weapon in Mother Nature's Army is another must for your shopping list.

Beetroot is a good source of iron and folate and contains nitrates, betaine, magnesium, vitamin C and fibre, which all have a beneficial effect on health.

Although eating cooked beetroot is good for you, the best way to ingest this potent vegetable is to drink its pressed, pure juice. This way all of its nutrients are intact (with the exception of fibre), as cooking will lose vitamin C.

BEET JUICE: It is early days in regard to research into beet juice, but scientists are intrigued by initial tests showing health benefits to blood pressure and blood flow throughout the body, including the brain, heart and muscles. There is strong evidence to show that it can boost exercise performance and help prevent dementia.

Beet juice is believed to relieve many diseases related to calcification in the body, like arthritis, heart disease, cancer, kidney stones, eye problems and varicose veins.

The good news is that most supermarkets now stock cartons of pressed, organic beetroot juice, containing 90% beetroot juice and 10% apple juice. If you drink it through a straw you will avoid the risk of getting a red moustache! Be prepared also for your urine and stools to have a pink/reddish appearance.

In addition to cooked beetroot and beet juice, why not try grating or peeling raw beetroot onto your salad?

BELL PEPPERS

Bell peppers have a beautiful, plump, glossy appearance and come in a wide variety of colours. The sweetest and most popular being the yellow, orange and red peppers. These are all the same variety but at different stages of ripening. They are most abundant during the summer months and early autumn.

The most exciting thing about these colourful jewels is that studies have shown that they are extremely rich in vitamin C and carotenoid content, which increases with ripening, as does their flavour. At the same time their total antioxidant capacity increases too. However, cooking at high temperatures can damage some of the delicate plant nutrients in bell peppers. To take advantage of their potent nutrients it is better to eat them uncooked, on a salad, in a salsa or as a garnish. Light cooking for a short time is better than cooking at high temperatures.

A wide variety of health studies, specifically from bell peppers, are producing exciting expectations, including the prevention of cardiovascular disease and of type 2 diabetes. Other areas of expectation include benefits for eye health. This must surely be the tip of the iceberg!

Although research studies have tended to focus on carotenoids as the hallmark antioxidant in bell peppers, this gem of a vegetable also provides minerals such as iron, copper, zinc, potassium, manganese and selenium, together with a very impressive, broad range of antioxidants including:

Vitamins: Very rich source of Vitamin C – especially so in red peppers, Vitamin B Complex, vitamin E and Vitamin A (in the form of beta-carotene).

Flavonoids: Luteolin, quercetin and hesperidin.

Carotenoids: Alpha-carotene, concentrated amounts of beta-carotene, cryptoxanthin, lutein,

There is no doubt that bell peppers have a remarkable track record as an antioxidant rich food.

BLUEBERRIES

Blueberries are low in calories and pack a real antioxidant punch, having the highest antioxidant capacity of all fresh fruit. They also have anti-inflammatory, anti blood clotting and antibacterial effects.
.

After many years of research into blueberry antioxidants and their potential benefits for the nervous system and for brain health, there is also exciting evidence that blueberries can improve memory. Encouraging research is still going on into their cardiovascular and cancer prevention properties.

It is the many different pathways for cardio support that are so striking in the blueberry research. The types of cancer already extensively studied, in respect of blueberry intake, include breast cancer, colon cancer and cancers of the small intestine. We look forward to the results of large-scale human studies on the potential ability of blueberry intake to lower the risks of these cancer types.

Other health gains include blood sugar benefits for those with type 2 diabetes. In many cases, those diagnosed with obesity also face the challenge of maintaining a balanced blood sugar level (See Page 74).

BROCCOLI

Broccoli belongs to the potent cruciferous group of vegetables, also known as brassicas. The most common of which are Broccoli, Kale, Cabbage, Sprouts and Cauliflower. All are packed with health benefits.

According to the 'The World's Health Organisation' (WHO), Broccoli has some special cholesterol lowering benefits and has a strong, positive impact on our body's detoxification system. In addition, broccoli has anti-inflammatory benefits and, if a minimum of only two cups of broccoli twice per week is eaten, this would be enough to help provide cancer prevention benefits.

WHO also report that broccoli contains ample supplies of vitamin A (in the form of beta-carotene) and vitamin K, which are necessary to help keep our vitamin D metabolism in balance. Broccoli also offers digestive support as is contains approximately 1 gram of dietary fibre for every 10 calories! Few components of food support our digestive system as well as fibre.

Never overcook broccoli. Always lightly steam for no longer than five minutes for maximum nutrition and flavour. As the fibrous stems may require a little longer to cook, they can be prepared separately and cooked a few minutes before adding the florets.

Scientists are continuing to develop our understanding of what unique properties in broccoli makes it a particularly healthy food. Studies have shown that people with a high proportion of brassicas in their diet have lower risks of some diseases.

KIWI FRUIT

There is more vitamin C in a kiwi fruit than an equivalent amount of orange. This antioxidant is the primary source of water soluble vitamin in the body, neutralising free radicals that can cause damage to cells and lead to problems such as inflammation and cancer. Kiwi fruit is also rich in vitamin K. Smaller amounts of nutrients include vitamin E, folate and the minerals potassium and manganese. In addition they are a very good source of dietary fibre. Fibre has been shown to be useful for blood sugar control, plus cardiovascular and colon health.

Most people discard the skin of kiwi fruit but, in fact, this is edible and is rich in nutrients and fibre. The 'fuzz' can be rubbed off before eating. Do eat this fruit as soon as it is ripe (slightly soft to the touch) as the longer it is left the fewer nutrients it retains.

In the world of plant nutrient research, kiwi fruit has fascinated researchers for its ability to protect DNA from free radical damage. As this fruit contains a variety of flavonoids and carotenoids that have demonstrated antioxidant activity, it is thought that these nutrients may be responsible for the DNA protection.

NOTE: Individuals with existing and untreated kidney or gallbladder problems may want to avoid eating kiwi fruit due to it containing small amounts of oxalates. When oxalates become too concentrated in body fluids, they can crystallize and cause health problems.

ORANGES

Like Kiwi Fruit, Oranges are an excellent source of vitamin C, the primary water soluble antioxidant in the body, disarming free radicals – the bad guys. Vitamin C is vital for the function of a healthy immune system.

This sweet and juicy fruit is also an excellent source of dietary fibre. In addition, oranges are a good source of B vitamins, vitamin A (in the form of beta–carotene), calcium, copper and potassium.

According to the World's Healthiest Foods Organisation, an orange has over 170 different plant nutrients and more than 60 flavonoids, many of which have been shown to have anti inflammatory, anti tumour and blood clot inhibiting properties, as well as strong antioxidant effects.

CSIRO (Commonwealth Scientific & Industrial Research Organisation) has reported that citrus fruits are protective against overweight and obesity conditions, which increase the risk of heart disease, certain cancers, diabetes, high blood pressure and strokes.

Little wonder that oranges are one of the most popular fruits in the world.

Choose oranges that are firm and heavy for their size. These will have a higher juice content than those that are either spongy or lighter in weight.

Useful Tips:

- Place freshly squeezed orange juice in ice–cube trays until frozen, then store the frozen cubes in plastic bags in the freezer for later use.

- The zest of oranges should be stored in a cool, dry place in an airtight glass container.

- The zest is a good addition to a smoothie for a stronger flavour and added nutrients.

SPINACH

A true superfood. Spinach is a top ranking nutrient rich vegetable. It contains a wealth of nutrients including Vitamin A (in the form of Beta-Carotene), B1, B2, B3, B5, B6, folate and vitamin C. Also manganese, magnesium, iron, copper, calcium, potassium, phosphorus, zinc, omega 3 fats, selenium and fibre. No wonder spinach can claim a special place among vegetables in terms of its nutrients content.

No surprise that spinach helps to protect against inflammatory problems, cardiovascular problems, bone problems and some cancers.

Before cooking wash the spinach well. Unlike most vegetables, boiling is recommended to free up acids and allow them to leach into the boiling water. This brings out a sweeter taste from the spinach. Use a large pot with lots of water and bring to a rapid boil. Add the spinach to the boiling water and boil for not more than one minute. Begin timing as soon as you place the spinach in the pot if you are using less than 1.lb. of spinach. Discard the boiling water after cooking.

If you are serious about building a strong immune system by eating antioxidant rich foods to help combat free radicals, spinach has to be on your list of vegetables. You may not instantly have bulging muscles like Popeye but spinach will help to promote your wellbeing and vitality.

TOMATOES

MAN'S BEST FRIEND

Tomatoes are widely known for their outstanding antioxidant content, in particular their rich concentration of 'Lycopene'. This potent antioxidant has always been associated with its well researched ability to definitely help lower the risk of prostate cancer in men. Another key tomato plant nutrient which has received special focus in prostate cancer prevention is 'Alpha-tomatine'.

Along with prostate cancer and non-small cell lung cancer, pancreatic cancer and breast cancer are the best studied areas involving tomatoes and cancer risk.

Reduced risk of heart disease is another area of health benefits in which tomatoes truly excel. No body system has a greater need for antioxidant protection than the cardiovascular system. The heart and bloodstream are responsible for taking oxygen breathed in through the lungs and circulating it throughout the body. In order to keep oxygen in check, antioxidant nutrients are needed in abundance. It has to be noted that the conventional vitamins C and E provide added critical antioxidant support in the cardiovascular system.

Fresh tomatoes and tomato extracts have been shown to help lower total cholesterol and triglycerides (natural fats). In addition, tomato extracts have been shown to help prevent unwanted clumping together of platelet cells in the blood; a factor that is especially important in lowering the risk of heart problems like atherosclerosis.

But it doesn't stop there. Tomatoes have several other health benefits. In multiple studies, diets that include tomatoes have been linked with reduced risk of some

43

neurological diseases, including Alzheimers disease. In a few studies, tomato inclusive diets have also been linked with reduced risk of obesity.

Tomatoes are delicious cold in a salad but they are at their most potent when chopped and cooked in a little olive oil. This method releases more lycopene and beta-carotene from the skins. Cooking also tempers the acid and bitter qualities in tomatoes and brings out their warm, rich sweetness.

There are more potent, antioxidant rich fruits and vegetables which equal most of those on the top ten list. Here are a few others, in alphabetical order, which I would recommend you introduce into your healthy eating plan:

- Beans: Green & tinned varieties
- Berries such as raspberries, strawberries, blackberries and blackcurrants.
- Brussels Sprouts
- Cabbage
- Carrots
- Celery
- Cherries in season
- Garden Peas – fresh or frozen
- Kale
- Leeks
- Lemons and Limes
- Melons
- Pears
- Watercress

You now have the tools to help provide a healthy future. A healthy future is a happy one. However, there is a

'But'....you must also be aware of the four single most hazards which are likely to hijack your plan. These are......

- Free Radicals
- Too much sugar
- Too much saturated fat
- Too much salt

Chapters 5 and 6 will arm you with vital information in regard to WHY you must be on guard, every day, against the damage that too much sugar, saturated fats, salt and free radicals can cause.

He who ignores the powers of nutrition wastes the time of the physician
(Old Chinese Proverb)

He who ignores the powers of nutrition wastes the time of the physician
(Old Chinese Proverb)

PART 3

THE BAD GUYS

He who ignores the powers of nutrition wastes the time of the physician
(Old Chinese Proverb)

He who ignores the powers of nutrition wastes the time of the physician
(Old Chinese Proverb)

Chapter 5

FREE RADICALS – THE ENEMY

Free Radicals are toxins. It is the name given to substances that can interfere with, and damage, the living cells in your body. It is important to understand what causes free radicals. If you want to be healthy you cannot ignore the truth about the bad guys.

The following examples will give you a brief overview of how free radicals invade your cells every day of your lives. In so doing they may have the ability to break down your immune system, if not protected by antioxidants – the good guys! You will see that there are several sources of free radicals, most of which are out of your control as many are in the air you breathe such as…

- Air pollution caused by exhaust fumes
- Smoke from industrial plants
- Smoke from cigarettes
- Irritants in the air such as pesticides and insecticides

Apart from the toxins you inhale, the first port of call where you are likely to come into contact with free radicals, as far as the food chain is concerned, is on the skins of the fruits and vegetables you buy. It is likely that they have been exposed to components of free radicals such as pesticides, insecticides and pathogens (disease causing bacteria).

According to the Environmental Working Group (EWG), the fruits and vegetables with the most pesticides are apples, strawberries, grapes, celery, peaches, spinach, sweet bell peppers, imported nectarines, cucumbers, cherry tomatoes and potatoes. Their report states that a single grape sample contained 15 pesticides and the average potato had more pesticides, by weight, than any other food. You may find their web site interesting: www.ewg.org, particularly the EWG's Shoppers Guide to Pesticides.

To avoid being exposed to free radicals, you could make a habit of immersing all your newly purchased, fresh fruit into a clean bowl of cold water, with a few generous splashes of ordinary malt vinegar, for about ten minutes (You can buy a 2.lt container of malt vinegar from the supermarket for approximately £3.00), then drain and dry with a clean tea towel. You will notice the difference in the appearance of the fruit, it will shine and scream out to be eaten. Remember, a lot of nutrients are contained in the skins of fruit.

Note: Vinegar will act as a disinfectant, clearing any residue left on the surface of your fruit without leaving any taste. This also gives your fruit a longer shelf life.

Even burned particles on toast or on bits of food such as bacon, become free radicalised. When food is burned it completely alters the molecular structure of the food, making it an alien, un-natural form which invades our unsuspecting cells. If we did not have antioxidants to disperse the problem the cells would become damaged, which may trigger damaged cells to multiply, causing serious health problems.

Without ANTIOXIDANTS to diffuse free radicals, our defences would be down and the enemy would strike, so much so, that numerous infections and possibly cancers would occur within a few months. This is WHY eating a minimum of 'Six' pieces of fruit and vegetables (Two different fruits and four different vegetables) every day, is vital for building a healthy immune system. Try and aim for seven portions a day!

Note: All fruits and vegetables are a valuable source of fibre, which helps cleanse the system of toxins.

He who ignores the powers of nutrition, wastes the time of the physician
(Old Chinese Proverb)

He who ignores the powers of nutrition, wastes the time of the physician
(Old Chinese Proverb)

Chapter 6

SUGARS, FATS, SALT

Sugars

Sugar is addictive, often referred to as the heroin of the food chain. Recent research has deemed it to be Public Enemy Number One. It requires knowledge and discipline for us to cut back on our consumption. Any sugar that the body doesn't need is converted into fat which leads to weight gain.

All sugars are high in calories. There are bad sugars and 'Not as bad'' sugars. I cannot describe 'sugar' as being good because sugar is not good; there are some sugars that are worse than others!

<u>Bad Sugars</u>: When any type of sugar is added to foods during cooking, processing or at the table, you consume calories without any nutrients or fibre. This type of sugar is referred to as 'added sugar', which is bad sugar. We all know the temptation of consuming foods with added sugar such as cakes, biscuits, sweets, ice cream, jams, soft drinks and table sugar. However, refined /added sugars are hidden in many savoury food products too, in an effort to satisfy the pallet of the developed world's population! Without realising it we are getting sugar overload, relying on our pancreas to work overtime by releasing enough insulin to deal with its metabolism within our bodies.

<u>'Not as Bad'Sugars</u>: Known as 'Simple Sugars', the main ones being 'Glucose & Fructose'.

<u>Glucose</u> occurs naturally in fruits, vegetables, nuts and whole grains. When simple sugars are naturally found in whole foods, apart from their antioxidant properties, they also come armed with the all important ingredient, fibre, which slows down the absorption of sugar into the bloodstream.

<u>Fructose</u> consists of approximately half glucose and half fructose. It occurs naturally in fruit and some vegetables and especially in honey. Of all foods, honey has the most dense concentrate of fructose. It is the sweetest sugar known, therefore it is very high in calories and should be avoided if you are trying to lose weight. Otherwise use infrequently and sparingly.

It is important not to be tempted by 'sweet, comfort foods' but they can be eaten infrequently and in small amounts as part of a balanced diet.

In the case of obesity and the dangers of diabetes 2, the hormone 'Insulin' is required to process, i.e. metabolise, glucose. Diabetes is a metabolic disorder which reduces the ability of the body to control the amount of glucose in the blood. Most carbohydrates in food are ultimately converted into glucose during digestion, so be mindful of how much carbohydrate you have in your diet.

Fructose, however, does not rely on insulin for its metabolism. The liver is the only organ that can metabolise fructose in significant amounts.

Some bad news regarding Fructose is that recent research is revealing that too much consumption of fructose may potentially have dangerous consequences for the liver, the arteries and the heart. Preliminary studies by Yale University have found that fructose may stimulate appetite.

Remember, fructose is a natural sugar and any 'processed' fructose' for use in alternative products, should definitely be avoided, in particular high-fructose corn syrup.

F A T S

All fats are very high in calories so it is important to bear this in mind if you are watching your weight. However, our bodies need fat to help it work normally. The important message is to swap saturated fats for unsaturated fats. Too much saturated fat can increase the amount of cholesterol in the blood, which can increase the risk of developing coronary heart disease, heart attacks and strokes.

BAD FATS: Saturated fats are in all animal fats and animal bi-products like butter, ghee, cheese and lard, all high in cholesterol. Other fats to avoid are trans fats and palm oils.

Avoid trans fats (trans fatty acids) wherever possible. Processed trans fats can be formed when oil goes through a process called hydrogenation, which makes the oil more solid. This type of fat, known as hydrogenated fat, is most likely to be found in processed foods such as biscuits, cakes, pastries and deep fried foods.

The most worrying thing about trans fats is that there are currently no legal requirements for food manufacturers to label 'trans fats'. This means that you need to check ingredient lists for trans fats, hydrogenated fats or hydrogenated vegetable oils.

<u>GOOD FATS</u>: The fats which are better for your health are those with a high monounsaturated oil content. These are olive oil, rapeseed oil and groundnut oil, as well as some nuts and seeds.

Foods with a high concentrate of monounsaturated fats include avocados, nuts, olives and oily fish such as salmon, trout, mackerel and sardines. I would highly recommended that you include this range of foods into your balanced diet routine, particularly avocado, sardines and salmon.

Olive Oil: Olive oil is rich in antioxidants, especially vitamin E. It contains the highest amount of monounsaturated oil than any other plant oil.

This oil is only suitable for cooking at low temperatures as it does not have the same high heat tolerance as other culinary oils. However, it is very good for salad dressings, marinades and gentle cooking methods and, according to the experts, it has many added health benefits due to its high antioxidant content, including cardiovascular disease.

Rapeseed Oil: According to Wharfe Valley Farms in West Yorkshire, producers of Cold Pressed Rapeseed Oil, this oil has the lowest saturated fat of any culinary oil and less than half that of Olive Oil.

Rapeseed Oil remains stable at high temperatures, is high in monounsaturated fats and is trans fat free. It also contains vitamin E.

Groundnut Oil is made from peanuts. It is high in monounsaturated fats and, unlike olive oil, it tolerates

high temperatures as does rapeseed oil. Groundnut oil is also a natural source of antioxidants including vitamin E.

Groundnut oil should be avoided if you have a nut allergy.

Polyunsaturated fats help to maintain healthy cholesterol levels and provide essential fatty acids. These fats are found in soya, vegetable and sunflower oils and spreads made from these oils, oily fish and some nuts and seeds such as walnuts and sesame seeds.

Remember, good fats can be healthy if small amounts are used in moderation as part of a balanced diet.

Omega-3 Fatty Acids: These are polyunsaturated fatty acids that are essential nutrients for health, their most crucial role arguably being in the prevention of cardiovascular diseases like heart attacks and strokes.

According to Dr. Frank Sacks, Professor of Cardiovascular Disease Prevention at Harvard School of Public Health, you should aim to get at least one rich source of Omega-3 Fatty Acids in your diet every day. This could be through a serving of fish, such as salmon, a handful of walnuts or ground flaxseeds mixed into your morning oatmeal or porridge.

Other sources of Omega-3 Fatty Acids include avocado, cauliflower, Brussels Sprouts and mustard seeds.

SALT

The GDA (Guideline Daily Amount) of salt for adults is 6g per day - that's about one level teaspoon.

You might be surprised how much hidden salt there is in everyday foods, particularly processed foods, such as cereals, breads, biscuits and cakes. If you eat these foods often the amount of salt you are eating can really add up. Even the salt you add during cooking counts towards your GDA. In fact, around three quarters of the salt you eat has already been added to your food before you buy it. So the level teaspoon GDA leaves you with one quarter of a teaspoon to add to your food at the table per day!

If you are using salt, I would recommend that you use unrefined, pink 'Himalayan' salt for its high mineral content. You will find it in your local health store.

Babies who are breastfed receive the right amount of sodium through breast milk, and infant formula is manufactured to contain a similar amount.

Suggestions on how to cut down on salt:

- Always taste your food first to see if it needs salt.

- Stop adding salt to your food during cooking.

- Stop or cut down on salt at the dinner table.

- On salads use balsamic vinegar and/or herbs such as mint, coriander, basil etc., for flavour.

- Cooked meals: Add herbs and spices instead of salt to flavour your food.

He who ignores the powers of nutrition wastes the time of the physician
(Old Chinese Proverb)

PART 3

THE GOOD

THE BAD

&

THE UGLY

He who ignores the powers of nutrition wastes the time of the physician
(Old Chinese Proverb)

He who ignores the powers of nutrition wastes the time of the physician
(Old Chinese Proverb)

Chapter 7

DRINKS

To stay healthy it's important to replace the fluids we lose when we breathe, sweat or urinate. Our bodies need water or other fluids to avoid dehydration. We get our fluid from all drinks and from food.

Signs of dehydration through not drinking enough fluids are:

- Headaches
- Lack of energy – feeling tired
- Feeling lightheaded
- Dark urine and not passing much urine.

The healthiest drinks are water and milk. A small glass of freshly pressed or squeezed fruit juice is also a healthy drink – add water if you are thirsty and require a large glass, this will avoid sugar overload.

Avoid soft and fizzy drinks that can be high in added sugars. These can be high in calories and bad for your teeth. Some energy drinks are high in both sugar and caffeine. It's wise to check the nutrition label on these drinks to help you make healthier choices.

WATER

Unless you are taking part in high endurance sports, water is the healthiest choice and the best way to quench your thirst and replace fluids lost through exercise.

Most of the chemical reactions that happen in your cells need water in order to take place. You also need water so that your blood can carry nutrients around the body and get rid of waste. In fact, water makes up about two-thirds of the weight of a healthy body!

To help revive you when fatigue sets in, drink a glass of water. If you don't like the taste of plain water try adding a slice of lemon or lime. You could also add a little pure fruit juice.

The European Food Safety Authority recommends that women should drink about 1.6 litres of fluid every day, (that's about 8 x 200ml glasses each day), and men should drink about 2.0 litres of fluid, (about 10 x 200ml glasses per day), to avoid becoming dehydrated. However this amount depends on a range of factors, including your size, the daily temperature and how active you are.

MILK

Milk contains more nutrients than any other single food.

Milk is a good source of calcium, which helps build and maintain healthy bones, vitamin B12 and other vitamins and minerals. It is also valuable for its protein content.

If you are getting enough 'fat' in your diet, choose either semi-skimmed,1% fat or skimmed milk. Limit your intake of flavoured milks, milkshakes, condensed milk and milk-based energy or malt drinks as these contain added sugar.

A coffee made with skimmed milk, mid morning, is a top tip to keep hunger pangs at bay 'till lunch time.

TEA

After water, tea is the most popular drink.

Black, green and white teas all come from the same plant, the Chinese Camellia Sinensis. All of these teas contain antioxidants and caffeine to varying degrees. The antioxidants in tea help protect against heart disease, strokes and cancer.

White tea comes from the buds and tender leaves of the plant. It is the purest of all teas and is richer in antioxidants than green and black tea due to the minimal amount of processing. It is much milder than other teas and contains little caffeine. It does, however, contain high levels of health promoting catechins (see 'Note' below).

Green tea is produced by a process which does not allow as much oxidation as black tea but, it does open the door for more caffeine to develop at the cost of a reduction in antioxidants. It has a more defined flavour than white tea.

It is thought that the antioxidant group of catechins and caffeine in green and white tea may have a role in helping the body burn more calories, sometimes referred to as 'Speeding up the metabolism', which can help with weight loss.

Note: 'Catechins' are a powerful group of plant-chemical antioxidants contained particularly in white and green tea. These have been found to reduce cholesterol, thereby improving the function of blood vessels and decreasing blood pressure, thus decreasing the risk of cardiovascular disease. Catechins also provide anti-inflammatory activities. They help in the prevention of vascular inflammation that plays a critical role in the progression of atherosclerotic lesions.

Black tea: Unlike white and green tea, black tea is strong in flavour and it retains its flavour for up to a year. It contains fewer antioxidants and more caffeine than white or green tea.

COFFEE

The jury is still not clear in regard to whether coffee is good or bad for you. This is because people vary in the way their bodies process the caffeine in coffee. Therefore, it could be bad for some but not for others! Also the variation in its processing methods plus roasting and brewing techniques, are all factors that can alter the taste and chemical makeup of the coffee.

It is well known that coffee is a stimulant due to the amount of caffeine it contains. I guess this is the reason why so many people like their coffee fix first thing in a morning! Coffee is a diuretic depending on how strong you make it and how much you drink.

According to The British Heart Foundation, a recent study has claimed that moderate consumption of coffee may reduce your risk of heart failure. However, more than four 150ml cups per day was found to increase peoples risk of heart failure! Remember, coffee shops offer coffee in much larger sizes, so be aware of the quantities you are drinking.

If you make your coffee with milk there is no need to add sugar as milk contains 'Lactose', its own form or sugar.

It is important that coffee or tea are not your only source of fluid.

FRUIT JUICES & SMOOTHIES

A 150 ml glass of pure fruit juice counts as one of your 'five a day' portions of fruit and vegetables. One small glass a day is sufficient. Fruit juices, particularly apple juice, is very high in sugar. I would recommend that you dilute your fruit juices with water if drinking more than a 150ml glass.

The sugar in fruit juice can damage teeth so it is better to drink it when having a meal or to drink it through a straw. However, the key issue as far as high sugar content in fruit juices and fizzy drinks is concerned, is the lack of fibre (see chapter 3). When we eat fresh fruit, particularly with the skin on, fibre forms a protective layer that acts as a barrier to the intestine. This slows the absorption of sugar into the bloodstream. In fruit drinks the barrier has gone due to the absence of fibre, which is not good for people with diabetes.

When purchasing fruit juice always check the label. Choose 100% pressed or squeezed fruit juice with no added sugar and not made from 'concentrate'.

Smoothies that are 100% fruit or vegetable count up to two portions towards your 'five a day' when they contain all the edible pulped fruit or vegetable. This also depends on the quantity and quality of the fruit and vegetables or juice used.

Any Juice drank in addition to a smoothie does not count as more towards your five a day portion.

FIZZY DRINKS & SQUASHES

Fizzy drinks and squashes contain very few nutrients and lots of sugar which means lots of calories. Calories contribute to weight gain. Cutting down or cutting out these drinks is a good way of reducing the number of calories you consume, while not missing out on the nutrients.

A good substitute for fizzy drinks is to add a good measure of sparkling water to natural fruit juices.

ALCOHOL

The following account of calories in alcohol is in accordance with 'Live Well' – NHS Choices.

Wine, beer, cider, spirits and all our favourite alcoholic drinks are made from natural starch and sugar. Fermentation and distillation for certain drinks is used to produce the alcohol content. This helps explain why alcohol contains lots of calories – seven calories per gram!! Remember, additional calories can be present in added mixer drinks.

In March 2009, an online survey was carried out in the UK by YouGov for the Department of Health. Nearly 2,000 people took part and the following findings were drawn from the results:

- The average drinker in England takes in around 2,000kcal from alcohol every month.

- Drinking five pints of lager a week adds up to 44,200kcal over a year, equivalent to eating 221 doughnuts!

- A heavy drinking session is often followed by an unhealthy breakfast to help cope with a hangover, which again helps to pile on the pounds. Going for a fry-up instead of your usual bowl of cereal can add an extra 450kcal to the calorie count from the night before.

- Many drinkers add to their calorie intake by having snacks, such as crisps, nuts or pork scratchings, to accompany their tipple.

- Many women don't realise that two large glasses of white wine provides them with nearly 20% of their recommended daily calorie intake, at approximately 370kcal in total. It also puts them over the recommend daily limit for regular alcohol consumption.

- Regularly drinking too much alcohol can have a noticeable impact on your waistline and may cause less obvious but more serious health problems.

The NHS Recommends:

- Men should not regularly drink more than 3-4 units of alcohol a day
- Women should not regularly drink more than 2-3 units a day
- If you have had a heavy drinking session, avoid alcohol for 48 hours.

'Units' are a simple way of expressing the quantity of pure alcohol in a drink. One unit equals 10ml or 8g of pure alcohol, which is about the amount of alcohol an average adult can process in an hour. This means that within an hour there should be, in theory, little or no alcohol left in the blood of an adult, although this will vary from person to person.

The units in a drink are based on the size of the drink as well as its alcohol strength. For example...

- A pint of strong lager contains 3 units of alcohol, whereas the same volume of standard lager has just over 2 units.

- A small glass of red/white/rose wine contains 1.5 units

- A standard glass of red/white/rose wine contains 2.1 units.

- A large glass of red/white/rose wine contains 3 units.

Tips to avoid weight gain as recommended by the British Nutrition Foundation:

- Alternate an alcoholic drink with a glass of water. This will help to prevent you becoming dehydrated.

- Do not drink on an empty stomach. Snack on a healthy sandwich rather than reaching for the peanuts, crisps, chips or pork scratchings.

- Drink at your own pace, do not be drawn into drinking in rounds as this can mean you drink more than you intended.

- Pace yourself by taking small sips

- Try cutting down with a friend. With a bit of moral support you are more likely to stick to it.

- Avoid binge drinking.

Remember, calories from drinking alcohol soon add up.

He who ignores the powers of nutrition wastes the time of the physician
(Old Chinese Proverb)

He who ignores the powers of nutrition wastes the time of the physician
(Old Chinese Proverb)

Chapter 8

EATING A BALANCED DIET

<u>PROTEIN</u>

Protein is an important part of a healthy balanced diet. It is essential for the healthy growth and repair of all your body tissues, such as your muscles (including your heart) and internal organs, such as your lungs, liver, and skin. Protein is also an important source of energy for the body when carbohydrates and fats are not available.

Excellent sources of protein include turkey, tuna, shrimp and cod.

Very good sources of protein include halibut, salmon, scallops, sardines, chicken, lamb, grass-fed beef, liver, spinach, tofu, asparagus, soybeans, cheese and nuts.

Good sources of protein include eggs, squash, cauliflower, lentils, kidney beans, black beans and pinto beans.

Experts from the Harvard School of Public Health and Harvard Medical School, encourage limiting red meat and avoiding processed meat, since eating even small quantities of these foods on a regular basis raises the risk of heart disease, diabetes, colon cancer and weight gain.

-0-0-0-

CARBOHYDRATES

The main function of carbohydrates is to provide energy to your body and brain. When ingested it is broken down into glucose, which is absorbed into the bloodstream for the utilisation of energy to your muscles and other tissues.

Main sources of carbohydrate are starchy foods such as potatoes, bread, cereals, rice and pasta. Wholegrain varieties, particularly potatoes with their skins on, provide good sources of fibre. However, potatoes are full of rapidly digested starch and can have the same effect on blood sugar as refined grains and sweets, so I would recommend that you limit your consumption, particularly if you are diabetic.

Starchy foods contribute to a range of nutrients in your diet. As well as starch they contain fibre, calcium, iron and 'B' vitamins. Their calorie content is half that of fat. However, the calorie content would be increased by added fat when cooking and serving, for example putting mayonnaise on a baked jacket potato, spreading butter on bread or eating egg fried rice instead of boiled rice. Moderation and quantity is key when adding fat if you are watching your weight.

Experts from the Harvard School of Public Health and Harvard Medical School have advised that refined grains, like white bread and white rice, act just like sugar. Eventually, eating too much of these refined-grain foods can make it harder to control weight and can raise the risk of heart disease and diabetes.

–0–0–0–

Government Guidelines

Government guidelines on dietary advice for people who are obese and/or diabetic are similar to that for the population in general, i.e. maintenance of a healthy weight and consumption of a diet that is:

- low in sugars
- low in salt
- low in fat (particularly saturated fat)
- high in fruit and vegetables
- high in starchy carbohydrate foods, especially wholegrain types such as bread, chapatti, brown rice, pasta and yams. (I would question the 'High'! – See Page 72).

The Eatwell Plate has been published by the British Heart Foundation in accordance with the Food Standards Agency. However, due to a comprehensive review of the government's current guidelines on The Eatwell Plate, this has not been referenced in my book. Potentially the current information in regard to The Eatwell Plate may be superseded in a revised format by 'Public Health England' (PHE), which is due to be published in late Spring 2015. For information on the current UK guidelines you can go online to: www.gov.uk/the-eatwell-plate

MyPlate

The American equivalent of The Eatwell Plate is MyPlate.

This is the current nutrition guide published by the United States Department of Agriculture.

MyPlate is divided into sections of approximately 30% grains, 40% vegetables, 10% fruits and 20% protein, accompanied by a smaller circle representing dairy, such as a glass of milk or a yogurt cup.

These amounts are not meant to represent the portion-type balance required in any one specific meal, or over a particular timescale, rather they represent the overall balance of a healthy diet. Nor do they refer to frequency of serving or recommended portion sizes.

MyPlate has made additional recommendations, such as "Switch to 1% milk or skimmed milk", "Make at least half of your grains whole" and "Vary your protein food choices". The guidelines also recommend portion control while still enjoying food, as well as reductions in sodium and sugar intakes.

Blood Sugar Swings

Blood sugar swings are typical of a bad eating regime caused by habitual quick fix snacking on food, such as biscuits, cake and chocolate. It isn't long before energy levels stoop leaving you feeling tired and depleted. It will take discipline to get your blood sugar levels balanced. The sooner you start to eat properly, the sooner you will feel better.

This problem is caused by the level of blood glucose rising quickly after eating too much sugary foods, leaving the hormone, insulin, to release more than it would normally, this is followed by the level of blood sugar swinging low again.

Sometimes blood sugar swings can cause a feeling of shaking inside and a desperate need for something sweet. In this case a small, fresh apple or banana would be a far better choice than a chocolate bar or other sweet alternative. On occasions when for some reason you cannot eat your lunch until later in the day, it would be wise to take a banana or a small apple and a few nuts out with you to snack on.

Blood sugar swings can have an impact on your concentration and energy levels.

The best way to address low blood sugar swings is to eat a balanced diet at REGULAR INTERVALS – NO SKIPPING MEALS and by keeping sugary foods in check! Especially so for those with diabetes.

Eating a balanced diet is an important part of managing diabetes. If you have diabetes your blood glucose levels will be monitored by healthcare professionals, however, this can be done by yourself.

He who ignores the powers of nutrition wastes the time of the physician
(Old Chinese Proverb)

He who ignores the powers of nutrition wastes the time of the physician
(Old Chinese Proverb)

Chapter 9

INVEST IN YOUR HEALTH

Shopping for food is the starting point for investing in your health. What you put into your trolley on a regular basis will determine how healthy your future will be.

Remember, being overweight is generally caused by consuming more calories than you burn off through physical activity throughout your day, particularly those calories in fatty and sugary foods.

<u>Shopping lists</u>

To begin with here are a few shopping tips.

- When purchasing fruit and vegetables, always select the loose items and bag them yourself rather than the already packaged ones. You will find that this usually works out much cheaper too.

- When purchasing fresh fruit and vegetables, look for the ones that are firm and crisp. In most cases, if you wash and dry your fruit as soon as you get home (see page 50), it will keep longer and remove any free radicals.

- Buying organic is more expensive. You can always choose the organic option when you are able to make savings in other areas. It is more important to purchase organic root vegetables like carrots, celery and potatoes. Organic fruits and vegetables have more flavour, as do organic breads and soups.

- Look out for offers, particularly on those foods which you can freeze like salmon.

- Avoid purchasing processed food. Lots of meals made with fresh food are quick, easy and delicious. Meals, such as casseroles, soups and pies, can be made the day before or frozen. Try to plan ahead to avoid the quick fix, processed food option.

The following brief shopping lists include items for your weekly shop and for your store cupboard. Some items are not cheap but investing in your health should be considered when making choices.

Foods to include on your weekly/bi-weekly shopping list

Apples
Apricots in season
Avocados
Beetroot Juice: Small Carton
Bell Peppers –   Red Orange and/or Yellow
Berries of choice
Bread/Wholemeal
Fish –   Salmon, Trout, Smoked Mackerel or
                         other fish of choice
Green Vegetables: Broccoli, Cabbage, Courgettes,
                         Green Beans, Kale, Spinach, etc.,
Herbs for flavouring: Mint, Coriander, Basil, chives etc.,
Kiwi Fruit
Lemons
Meat: Chicken and/or other of choice

Nuts   Almonds, Brazils, Walnuts etc.,
Olives
Oranges
Organic: Carrots, Celery & Potatoes etc.,
Organic;   Milk & Bread
Pasta/Fresh
Pears
Rice/Wholemeal
Salad ingredients of choice
Tomatoes

Foods for your Store Cupboard

Garlic
Organic: Oats. Stock Cubes
Oils: Groundnut, Rapeseed or Sunflower
                        Oil, Olive Oil
Pasta/Dried
Rice – Wholegrain
Seeds: Sunflower, Pumpkin, Sesame
Spices...   Tumeric, ginger etc.,
Tea: Black, Green or White
Tins: Sardines, Pilchards, Salmon & Tuna.
                        Baked Beans, Organic Tomato Soup,
                        Sweet Corn, Tomatoes
Tomato Ketchup
Tomato Pure
Vinegar: Malt, Balsamic, Cider

−0−0−0−

Exercise

A healthy, balanced diet should go hand in hand with exercise. Some of us require more than others but it is important to get regular exercise, e.g. jogging, walking, swimming or cycling for at least one hour, three times per week. Or aim for half an hour five or six days a week.

If you don't like exercising alone, join a rambling or cycling club. Join a gym or arrange walks with a neighbour or friend.

It's all about getting into the habit. The hardest part is the first step – going out and doing it! Each time after that it becomes easier and more enjoyable, particularly when you start to see results.

Useful Tips

Lemon Drink:
Start each day with a cup of warm water that has been boiled and add the squeezed juice of half a lemon. We tend to think of lemons as 'acid' fruits which, indeed, they are but, when lemon juice is ingested it has an alkalising affect on our stomach and provides a terrific start to the day. The full explanation for this is based in biological science which can be sourced on line.

Organic Food:
Milk contains more nutrients than any other single food and, in my opinion, the extra cost incurred in buying organic milk is far outweighed by the great value you get from its health benefits. Also buy organic vegetables whenever possible.

WASH YOUR FRUIT: Wash and dry your fresh fruit to remove any pathogens, pesticides or insecticides before eating.

PORTIONS: Try to cut down on your portion sizes if trying to lose weight.

SLOW DOWN: Take more time eating your meal. The digestive track starts in your mouth where saliva juices begin to break down the food you eat.

HOBBIES: Often you can pick at comfort food out of boredom. If you have time on your hands start a new hobby such as painting, writing, reading, gardening, decorating, golf and/or other sports. Meet up with like minded friends every week for coffee or become a member of your local political party and join in their social functions.

Having a hobby and meeting people would focus your mind on other things and would help to stop you 'snacking'. Meal times would become more enjoyable.

THE FOUR P's: The following page sets out a list of four challenges. These should be addressed until they become an automatic part of the way you think in regard to investing in your health. It's part of the 'Train your Brain' strategy to help you keep on track.

He who ignores the powers of nutrition wastes the time of the physician
(Old Chinese Proverb)

THE FOUR P's

POSITIVE THINKING

Accept the challenge and deal positively with your conscious 'Eating for Life' plan.

PLANNING

Plan your meals a day in advance.

Plan your shopping list.

PREPARING

Be mindful of ingredients and how you can nutritionally enhance a meal without adding salt, sugar or saturated fat.

PERSEVERANCE

Keep trying. It takes time to re-train your brain.

RESEARCH

There are many international research organisations who are dedicated to unravelling the hidden, powerful nutrients in the foods we eat. For example:

- The work into the amazing anti-asthma benefits of the humble apple. This fruit appears to be a remarkable, standout fruit in regard to asthma benefits (Page 33).

- High research expectations into Bell Peppers in regard to reducing the risk of diseases, including the prevention of cardiovascular disease and of type 2 diabetes (Page 36).

- Beet juice is revealing qualities of health benefits to blood pressure and blood flow throughout the body including the brain, heart and muscles. There is also strong evidence to show that it can boost exercise performance and help prevent dementia (Page 35).

These examples are just the tip of the iceberg when it comes to research in the complex science of nutrition.

We must start to think differently about the food we eat and stop taking our food for granted.

He who ignores the powers of nutrition wastes the time of the physician
(Old Chinese Proverb)

GLOSSARY

Antioxidants Vital protective components found in food nutrients, particularly vitamins. Vitamins are mainly found in fruits and vegetables.

Calcification The accumulation of salts in body tissue.

Carcinogen A substance that can induce cancer.

Carotenoids A general term for the wide variety of organic red and yellow compounds that are found in plant foods, some of which the body can convert into vitamin A. Carotenoids are powerful antioxidants.

Dietary Fibre Material mainly derived from plant cell walls, most of which is not digested by human digestive enzymes.

Diuretic Adjective: Causing increased passing of urine. Noun: A diuretic drug.

Enzyme A protein that speeds up (catalyses) a metabolic reaction.

Flavonoids Plant based compounds best known for their antioxidant and anti-inflammatory properties.

Free Radicals	Toxins. Substances that can interfere and damage living cells in the human body.
GDA	Guideline Daily Amount.
HDL	High-Density Lipoproteins. These are the good fats which help reduce cholesterol levels.
LDL	Low-Density Lipoproteins. These are the bad fats that increase cholesterol levels.
Lipids	Dietary fats and oils.
Metabolism	The chemical process and reaction, and related reactions, that break down organic matter in our cells after digesting food, which is converted into energy to keep us alive.
Pathogens	Disease causing bacteria
Phytochemicals	Plant Chemicals. 'Phyto' is the Greek name for Plant.
Phytonutrients	Plant Nutrients. 'Phyto' is the Greek name for Plant.
Triglycerides	Main constituents of natural fats and oils

He who ignores the powers of nutrition wastes the time of the physician
(Old Chinese Proverb)

ACKNOWLEDGEMENTS

British Heart Foundation
CSIRO (Commonwealth Scientific & Industrial Research
Organisation) - www.csiro.au
Department of Health, Extracts from 'Manual of Nutrition' 12th
edition
Environmental Working Group - www.ewg.org
George Mateljan Foundation/The World's Healthiest Foods -
www.whfoods.org
Harvard University:
Harvard School of Public Health
Harvard T.H. Chan School of Public Health
Harvard School of Public Health, Department of Nutrition - Dr.
Frank Sacks, Professor of Cardiovascular Disease Prevention.
Harvard Medical School
National Institute of Health/extracts articles/PMC2748751
NHS Choices
The European Food Standards Agency
Wharfe Valley Farm, West Yorkshire

He who ignores the powers of nutrition, wastes the time of the physician
(Old Chinese Proverb)

JOURNAL

Train Your Brain

This section is for you to make notes as you read through the guide–book.

If you have a specific health issue you may want to log any relevant information which may help you.

You may also find it helpful to record page numbers which are of particular interest, or make general notes in regard to your progress etc.,

He who ignores the powers of nutrition, wastes the time of the physician
(Old Chinese Proverb)

He who ignores the powers of nutrition, wastes the time of the physician
(Old Chinese Proverb)